HOW TO OVERCOME AMENORRHEA

Best Natural Tips To Treat Scanty Periods

Theresa Abraham

Table Of Content

Chapter 1

ABOUT AMENORRHEA

Amenorrhea is missing one or more periods. If you are older than 15 and haven't had your first period (primary amenorrhea) or you've missed a period for a few months (secondary amenorrhea), speak to your healthcare practitioner. Amenorrhea is typically the symptom of a curable disease. Following therapy, your normal menstrual cycle will generally return.

What Is Amenorrhea?
Amenorrhea is when you don't receive your monthly period. It might be transient or permanent. Amenorrhea may develop from a change in function or a malfunction with some portion of the female reproductive system.

There are periods when you're not intended to receive your period, such as before puberty, during pregnancy, and after menopause. If amenorrhea lasts for more than three months, it should be explored.

How Does The Menstrual Cycle Work?
A complicated system of hormones governs the menstrual period. Every month, hormones prepare the body for pregnancy. Ovulation then occurs. If there is no pregnancy, the cycle concludes with the uterus losing its lining. Shedding is the menstrual cycle.

The hormones responsible for this cycle originate in diverse regions of the body. A malfunction in any of these organs may prevent a person from receiving a period:

Hypothalamus regulates the pituitary gland. The pituitary gland termed "the master gland" generates the hormones that direct the ovaries to ovulate.

Ovaries generate the egg for ovulation and the hormones estrogen and progesterone.
The uterus reacts to the hormones and prepares the lining. This lining sheds during the menstrual cycle if there's no pregnancy.

What Are The Forms Of Amenorrhea?
There are two categories of amenorrhea:
Primary amenorrhea is when you haven't obtained a first period by age 15 or within five years after the earliest indications of puberty. It might arise owing to changes in organs, glands, and hormones connected to menstruation.
Secondary amenorrhea is when you've been receiving regular periods, but you stop getting your period for at least three months, or you halt your menses for six months when they were previously irregular. Reasons might include pregnancy, stress, and sickness.

Who Is At Risk For Amenorrhea?
Risk factors for amenorrhea include:

Family history of amenorrhea or early menopause.
The genetic or chromosomal issue that impacts your menstrual cycle.
Obesity or being underweight.
Eating disorder.
Over-exercising.
Bad diet.
Stress.

Symptoms And Causes
What causes amenorrhea?
The various kinds of amenorrhea have distinct causes.

Frequent causes of primary amenorrhea include:
The chromosomal or genetic issue with the ovaries (the female sex organs that hold the eggs).
Hormonal concerns originate from abnormalities with the hypothalamus or the pituitary gland.

Structural difficulty with the reproductive organs, such as missing elements of the reproductive system.

Frequent causes of secondary amenorrhea include:
  pregnancy (which is the most prevalent cause of secondary amenorrhea).
Breastfeeding.
Menopause.
Certain birth control techniques, such as Depo Provera, intrauterine devices (IUDs), and some birth control tablets.
Chemotherapy and radiation treatment for cancer.
Prior uterine surgery with subsequent scarring (for example, if you had a dilation and curettage, frequently termed D&C).

Additional causes of secondary amenorrhea might include :
Stress
Inadequate nutrition.

Weight changes — severe weight reduction or obesity.
Exercise is connected with low weight.
Ongoing disease or chronic illness.

You may also have disorders that might induce secondary amenorrhea:
Primary ovarian insufficiency is when you undergo menopause before age 40.
Hypothalamus abnormalities, such as functional hypothalamic amenorrhea (FHA) — which is also termed hypothalamic amenorrhea (HA). FHA is a situation when amenorrhea is related to stress or weight loss, but isn't caused by an inherent problem with a woman's biology.
Pituitary problems, such as benign pituitary tumors or excessive production of prolactin.
Other hormonal abnormalities, such as polycystic ovarian syndrome, adrenal diseases, or hypothyroidism.
Ovarian tumors.
Surgery to remove the uterus or ovaries.

What Are The Signs Of Amenorrhea?
The major symptom is the absence of menstruation. Additional symptoms depend on the reason. You may experience:
Hot flashes.
Nipples gushing milk.
Vaginal dryness.
Headaches.
Vision changes.
Acne.
Abundant hair growth on your face and body.

Diagnose And Tests
How is amenorrhea diagnosed?
If you miss a period, contact your healthcare practitioner. Your physician will question you about your symptoms and medical history. If amenorrhea developed due to pregnancy, you may start prenatal treatment. If it's occurring due to menopause, there is aid if symptoms are bothersome. Missing periods leading to menopause commonly begin in your 40s.

Your physician will do a physical assessment and a pelvic exam.

Will I Need Any Tests To Diagnose Amenorrhea?

Your healthcare practitioner may wish to conduct several tests, including:

Pregnancy test.

Blood tests evaluate hormone levels and diagnose thyroid or adrenal gland diseases.

Genetic tests, if you have primary ovarian insufficiency and are younger than 40. MRI, if your clinician detects an issue with the pituitary gland or hypothalamus.

Do I Need To Keep Track Of When My Periods Happened?

Diagnosing amenorrhea may be tricky. If the reason for amenorrhea isn't evident, such as pregnancy, your provider may urge you to maintain a record of changes in your menstrual cycle. This history of your periods might assist your physician to figure out a diagnosis.

Using an app or a notebook, note:\sHow long your periods last.
When you had your last menstruation.
Medicines you are taking.
Changes in your diet or workout routine.
Emotional issues you're facing, such as stress.

Management And Treatment
How is amenorrhea treated?
If your period ended due to menopause or pregnancy, your physician will not need to treat it. In other circumstances, your therapy will depend on the reason and may include:

Reducing weight by diets and exercise (if excess weight is the reason) .
Gaining weight with a tailored food plan (if excessive weight loss is the reason).
Stress management strategies.
Varying exercise levels.

Hormone therapy (medication), as recommended by your healthcare professional.
Surgery (in rare situations).

In addition, your healthcare professional may offer various therapies to aid with the adverse symptoms of amenorrhea:
Estrogen treatment to reduce hot flashes and vaginal dryness.
Calcium and vitamin D tablets help keep bones healthy.
Strength training.
Amenorrhea may be a sign of anorexia nervosa, an eating condition. If you or a loved one has this illness, speak to a healthcare expert immediately so you can obtain the correct treatment.

Will I Need Surgery For Amenorrhea?
Surgery for amenorrhea is uncommon. Your healthcare professional may suggest it if you have:
Genetic or chromosomal disorders.

Pituitary tumor.
Uterine scar tissue.

Prevention
How can I avoid amenorrhea?
Maintaining a healthy lifestyle may help avoid certain causes of secondary amenorrhea. Strive to:
Maintain a healthy weight and consume a nutritious diet.
Be conscious of your menstrual cycle (so you'll know if you miss a period).
Have frequent gynecological checkups, including getting a pelvic exam and Pap test.
Obtain regular and enough sleep.

Outlook
Will my menstruation return?
Normally, your period will return after you address the underlying problem. Nevertheless, it may take time to become regular again.

In certain situations, you may have a health condition that means you'll never get a period. If such is the case, your provider may speak to you about reproductive alternatives if you choose to have a kid.

Are There Complications Of Amenorrhea?
Amenorrhea is not life-threatening. Nevertheless, certain factors may lead to greater hazards over the long term, therefore amenorrhea should always be addressed. Researchers have observed an increased incidence of hip and wrist fractures in persons with amenorrhea. You may also be at increased risk for bone weakening and reproductive issues.

What Are The Consequences For Individuals With Amenorrhea?
Your result will depend on the reason. For example, if you have PCOS, you will likely require lifetime treatment to avoid health issues and to create regular periods.

Living With Amenorrhea

How can I take care of myself if I have amenorrhea?

Amenorrhea may damage bone health. It's crucial to consume a calcium-fortified diet and exercise frequently.

When Should I Visit My Healthcare Provider Regarding Amenorrhea?

You should notify your healthcare practitioner if you miss three months of periods or miss a period and:

Having difficulties with balance, coordination, or vision, which might suggest a more severe issue.

Generate breast milk when you have not given birth.

Observe excessive body hair growth.

Are older than 15 and haven't received your first period yet.

Chapter 2

SPICES AND HERBS TO TREAT SCANTY PERIODS

There are several efficient natural ideas and cures to manage scanty periods at home without any negative effects.

1. Nigella Seeds Powder With Honey
Combine 500 grams of nigella seeds powder with 50 grams of honey to form a thick paste. Consume 1 teaspoon 2-3 times daily with warm water to cure scanty periods without any adverse effects.

2. Carom Seeds And Nigella Seeds
Make a fine powder with an equal number of carom and nigella seeds. Every day take half a teaspoon of this with one cup of lukewarm milk before bedtime. One of the greatest solutions to cure scanty periods within one month.

3. Fenugreek Seeds, Sesame Seeds, And Jaggery Powder

Fenugreek seeds powder ½ teaspoon, ½ teaspoon of sesame seeds powder, and 1 teaspoon of jaggery powder. Boil them in one cup of water until it is ¼ cup. Use it every day for two to three weeks to manage your periods naturally.

4. Fenugreek And Sesame With Honey

Take fenugreek and sesame seeds in equal numbers and boil them in one glass of milk for 5-6 minutes then add 1 teaspoon of honey to it. Take it every day throughout periods for a better and more rapid outcome.

Fenugreek and sesame seeds are highly beneficial for scanty periods. It is also quite good for individuals confronting the issue related to anemia.

5. Black Cardamom, Cinnamon, And Dried Ginger

Mix 1 tablespoon of black cardamom powder, 2 teaspoons of cinnamon powder, and 4 tablespoons of dried ginger powder. Take ½ teaspoon with lukewarm water or milk early in the morning on an empty stomach and ½ teaspoon before retiring to bed every day for 2-3 weeks. Extremely effective to get rid of all reasons for scanty periods.

6. Mother-wort

This herb is extremely effective at lowering female internal reproductive organ symptoms, cramping, and female internal reproductive tone.

The mother-wort plant has been proven to softly stimulate the female internal organ, although furthermore assisting the female hormones with an efficiency that is beneficial in boosting blood flow.

7. Turmeric Powder, Sesame Seeds With White Butter

Shallow fry ½ teaspoon of turmeric powder, 1 teaspoon of sesame seeds in 1 teaspoon of white butter (Desi ghee), and rapidly add 1 cup of milk. Boil it for 2-3 minutes, you may put crushed almonds in it too. Turn off the stove and add 1 teaspoon of honey to it. Take it like tea, repeat 2-3 times daily to address scanty periods issue naturally.

8. Warm Milk With Clove And Almond Oil
Take one glass of warm water milk and blend 10-15 drops of clove oil with your regular meals. It may be a helpful therapy for poor or irregular blood flow. You may use 1 tablespoon of almond oil in warm milk to address this condition.

9. Salt And Water: Due to scanty periods you might experience considerable discomfort in the leg and lower abdomen region. In this scenario consume 1 teaspoon of salt with lukewarm water 3 times throughout the day. It will eliminate all

obstruction of blood and drain out illness
and toxins from the body.

Chapter 3

FRUITS TO TREAT SCANTY PERIODS

1. Papaya And Papaya Leaves Powder
Papaya is particularly beneficial for uterine and blood flow during periods. It also minimizes the causes of stress. Dried papaya leaves and crush them to a fine powder and take ½ teaspoon daily with lukewarm water 2 times a day. Extremely effective for this situation.

2. Grape Juice
Every day drink 5-6 teaspoons of fresh grape juice 2-3 times a day for one month routinely. Better to use red grape juice to address this condition. Better to use red grape juice to address this condition. In the following month, your issue will be fixed since red grapes are also great to improve the lower HB level or RBC level.

3. Mango Juice With Ginger Juice And Honey

Mango is one more great fruit to enhance blood flow during periods. Mix cow milk, 1 teaspoon of ginger juice, and 1 teaspoon of honey in one ripe mango pulp. Everyday usage of at least 2-3 glasses of mango juice to eliminate all the issues associated with scanty periods.

4. Mango Tree Bark

Mango tree bark is also beneficial to enhance blood flow during the menstrual cycle. If you are coping with scanty periods, take one inch of mango tree bark and boil it in one cup of water. When it becomes ¼ take it with one teaspoon of honey. Repeat this technique twice or thrice a day for speedy results. Start taking it 1 or 2 days before your period date.

5. Peach Flower

To make dry peach blossoms and produce a fine powder. Take 2 grams daily with lukewarm water. Best to cure scanty period issues naturally without any bad effects.

6. Banana Tree Leaves Ash
Prepare ash with banana leaves and ½ teaspoon with lukewarm water 2-3 times throughout the day. The finest to address scanty periods issue.

7. All Fruit Juices
Any fruit juice with vitamin C daily in your diet would eradicate all the reasons for scanty menstrual periods owing to weakness and Anemia.

Chapter 4

VEGETABLES TO TREAT SCANTY PERIODS

1. Carrot Leaves Water With Brown Sugar
Boil 1-2 fresh carrot leaves in 1 glass of water for 5-6 minutes and drain it. Allow it to cool and put 5-6 teaspoons of brown sugar in it and drink every day for one week. It will enhance blood flow and you might receive relief from bodily aches also.

2. Carrot Seeds With Jaggery Liquor
If a lady is suffering from this disease for a long time merely boil 1 gram of carrot Seeds and ½ gram of jaggery in 1 liter of water to create liquor. Consume this liquor throughout the day and maintain using it till the necessary outcome. This approach is also extremely good to minimize menstrual cramping.

3. Beetroot Leaves Powder With Aloe Vera Gel

Dry up beetroot leaves in the sun and produce a fine powder. Store it in a glass jar and everyday mix ¼ teaspoon of aloe vera gel to produce a sticky paste. Prepare a pill with it and take it with lukewarm warm water. Repeat this before going to sleep. Throughout one-month scanty periods, the issue will be cured naturally.

4. Radish Seeds

Radish Seeds are rich with critical vitamins and minerals that will enhance yours. Immune system and enhance blood circulation. They assist to cleanse the blood and wash out impurities and also protect you from illness.

Consume ½ gram of radish Seeds powder with lukewarm water every day till the necessary result

5. Lukewarm Onion Juice

Obtain fresh onion juice from shredding a medium size onion and boil it and drink 3 teaspoons 2-3 times throughout the day. Quick efficient natural advice to cure scanty periods of blockage.

6. Fenugreek Leaves Liquor
Consuming fenugreek leaves liquor is the greatest natural suggestion to address scanty periods issue quickly and naturally. Fenugreek provides protein, potassium, and vitamin C which are great to raise estrogen levels naturally. Several forms of female issues usually arise from uneven hormone levels.
The anti-inflammatory qualities of fenugreek are also effective to minimize inside-body inflammation. If you have scanty issues owing to uterine irritation then usage of fenugreek leaves liquor is the finest natural cure to the problem.

7. Ginger Tea With Salt And Bay Leaf

Ginger tea is deemed highly beneficial for the discomfort of menstruation. A natural ingredient in Ginger is highly good to promote blood flow and menstrual dysfunction. Bay leaves not only regulate scanty periods issues but also minimize discomfort produced by scanty menstrual. Add salt before consuming it for the best outcome.

8. Garlic Powder With Fennel Water

Take ½ teaspoon of garlic powder and mix it with lemon juice and create a paste, take it with fennel seed heated water 3 times a day. Found very much effective in scanty periods.

9. Ginger And Sugar Come Juice

Every day drink one glass of sugar cane with 2 teaspoons of fresh ginger juice for one month. The greatest and quick efficient techniques to cure scanty periods issue naturally.

Chapter **5**

NUTS AND DRY FRUITS FOR SCANTY PERIODS

All varieties of nuts and dry fruits are ideal to preserve your estrogen, progesterone, and testosterone levels to cure scanty periods. The fiber in nuts strengthens uterine walls and boosted blood levels.

1. Crushed Dried Fruits And Nuts
Grind walnuts, almonds, peanuts, pistachio, blackcurrants, sesame seeds, pumpkin seeds, and pine nuts in equal proportions. Put this in a glass container and take 1-2 teaspoons 4-5 times a day to address this condition permanently. Alternatively, boil 1 tablespoon of this combination in one of milk and eat it every day before going to bed.

2. Dried Figs

Boil 4-5 dried Figs in one glass of milk over low heat, after the liquid evaporates into one cup add 1 teaspoon of honey and sip as tea. Take 1-2 times throughout the day to address periods issue naturally.

3. Black Currants

Mash and boil 4-5 black currants in one glass of water on low heat, when it evaporates into one cup off the stove and put 1 teaspoon of honey in it. Consume it as tea 1-2 times a day. The best natural solution to cure scanty periods is naturally.

4. Almond And Walnuts Kernels With Jaggery Syrup

Prepare a thick syrup with 250 grams of jaggery and 125 ml water and set it to cool. Now add slightly crushed 250 grams of almond and walnut kernels and preserve it in a glass container. Every day take a teaspoon with one cup of warm milk for 2-3 months to cure scanty periods efficiently.

Chapter **6**

BEST SUPPLEMENT TO TREAT SCANTY PERIODS

Omega-3 Fatty Acids may aid fertility and increase the health of the ovary and origin. Oily fish like salmon and cod are excellent sources of Omega-3 fatty acids because Omega-3 fatty acids play a key function in hormone synthesis.

Omega-3 boosts your blood level and flow to heal scanty periods. Pumpkins, hemp, chia, and flax seeds are also packed with Omega-3 fatty acids, fiber, and oxidants, which increase the quality of blood by boosting ovarian health.

WHAT TO ADD AND WHAT TO AVOID

Hydrate your body with 8 glasses of filtered water every day since dehydration may aggravate the symptoms of scanty periods

Daily exercise might assist to open the clogged veins of the ovary and a healthy menstrual cycle.

Add zinc rich diet to regulate your hormonal level

Prevent to use of hot spicy dishes and junk foods

Increase the usage of garlic with daily meals

Strive to keep yourself stress-free since stress reduces your estrogen level which might create sexual health difficulties.

Add more estrogen-rich items to your diet every day

Incorporate additional Iron-rich meals into your everyday diet. The iron meal helps to generate more fresh blood in the body.